Natalia Montes Silva

Evidence for Occupational Therapy in Parkinson's Disease

Natalia Montes Silva

Evidence for Occupational Therapy in Parkinson's Disease

Evidence-based intervention proposal for the treatment of Parkinson's disease

ScienciaScripts

Imprint

Any brand names and product names mentioned in this book are subject to trademark, brand or patent protection and are trademarks or registered trademarks of their respective holders. The use of brand names, product names, common names, trade names, product descriptions etc. even without a particular marking in this work is in no way to be construed to mean that such names may be regarded as unrestricted in respect of trademark and brand protection legislation and could thus be used by anyone.

Cover image: www.ingimage.com

This book is a translation from the original published under ISBN 978-620-2-12736-3.

Publisher:
Sciencia Scripts
is a trademark of
Dodo Books Indian Ocean Ltd. and OmniScriptum S.R.L publishing group

120 High Road, East Finchley, London, N2 9ED, United Kingdom
Str. Armeneasca 28/1, office 1, Chisinau MD-2012, Republic of Moldova, Europe
Printed at: see last page
ISBN: 978-620-6-01809-4

Williard and Spackman (2009) explain that "Occupational Therapy is the art and science of helping people perform the activities of daily living that are important to their health and well-being through participation in valued occupations. Occupational therapy refers to all activities that occupy people's time and give meaning to their lives".

Evidence-based medicine (EBM) is the explicit and judicious use of the most effective evidence in making decisions about the care of individual patients. The term was coined in the 1980s by a group of Canadian internists and clinical epidemiologists at McMaster University, who, over the years, formed the Evidence-Based Medicine Working Group (1992).

Evidence-based medicine is characterised by the belief that: information derived from clinical experience and intuition can lead to erroneous conclusions if it is not solidly based on systematic observations; the study and knowledge of the basic theoretical mechanisms of disease is necessary but insufficient to guide clinical practice; and finally, the professional needs to know certain rules to rigorously evaluate the methodology used to obtain the scientific evidence on which to base decisions about a diagnosis or treatment.

EBM does not work on the basis of intuition, it says that through clinical experience and pathophysiology concrete clinical decisions can be made, emphasising the value of clinical examinations and scientific evidence provided for clinical research.

Evidence-based rehabilitation considers that rationality or biological effectiveness is not a test of clinical effectiveness, as it seeks to accelerate and improve the use in clinical practice of the best available evidence on a treatment.

People can present illnesses that make it impossible for them to have a good occupational performance, such as Parkinson's disease, which is a chronic illness that affects not only the person who suffers from it, but also their family and all those around them, thus involving a series of psycho-emotional, economic and social disorders, both for the person and their family. The course of the disease involves a series of feelings of sadness, despair, depression, anguish, anger and dissatisfaction with their lives that grow as the disease progresses; patients become ashamed of themselves, isolate themselves, causing problems with their families. Often when the disease progresses and becomes more aggressive, the person's partner takes on the role of caregiver, giving them an extra emotional burden, often affecting the relationship. This is where the

O.T. plays an important role in keeping the person active and able to be as independent as possible in their performance for as long as possible. It is for this reason that in the following manual, the importance of O.T. treatment in this disease and how it facilitates the person in their occupational performance to carry out their activities of daily living is made known; for this an exhaustive compilation of scientific studies through a systematic review that explain the importance of the same within this type of intervention is made; the reason for which it was decided to make this manual is that the field of O.T. is still unknown to some health professionals and it is not known for sure.O.T. is still unknown to some health professionals and it is not known for sure what is the role that is exercised in this area, therefore, through this manual seeks to demonstrate the role of occupational therapists and how important is O.T. for the lives of people so that they can perform correctly and independently in all occupations or activities they perform or wish to perform.

According to the National Institute of Statistics (INE, 2017) the Chilean population is ageing rapidly, there is greater dependence on older adults and an increase in participation in the informal labour market. Based on the 2017 CENSUS, the age group of older adults has increased considerably, having an increasing relevance in the total population of the country, reaching 11.4% in the over 60s with 1,717,478 people, the age group of 65 years and over is 1,217,576, corresponding to 8% of the population, highlighting the over 80s, which reach 14.7% with 250,840 people (Ministry of Health, 2010). On the other hand, Chile would increase its Demographic Dependency Index from 57.2 in 2005 to 60.0 in 2020.

According to the Geriatric and Gerontological Society of Chile (SEGG, 2015) more than 20% of people over 60 years of age suffer from some mental or neurological disorder. The Ministry of Health (MINSAL,

2017) indicates that the two main neurodegenerative diseases affecting older adults are Alzheimer's disease and Parkinson's disease, the latter being the most relevant for this manual.

In 1817, the English physician James Parkinson described what he called "shaking or trembling palsy", in which he reported six clinical cases characterised by trembling, festal gait with propulsion and slowness of movement. The monograph was not widely circulated at the time. It was Charcot who discovered what Parkinson reported and emphasised that the picture was not caused by paralysis and that not all patients had tremor. He highlighted bradykinesia and rigidity as the main symptoms. He also promoted the use of the name Parkinson's disease to honour the memory of the man who first described it.

Parkinson's is a chronic disease, which impairs the quality of life of sufferers and those around them (Chaná, 2010), as it affects the individual's functionality and expectations about their physical, social and mental well-being, which are fundamental components of health-related quality of life. They have various symptoms, including motor symptoms, which include bradykinesia, resting tremor, rigidity and altered postural reflexes (Rodríguez, et al., 2013). However, it is an even more complex syndrome which involves aspects that include cognitive disorders, sleep disorders, psychiatric disorders, oculomotor disorders, speech disorders, swallowing disorders, hypomimia (Chaná, 2010), and even involves a series of psycho-emotional, economic and social disorders (MINSAL, 2010).

Worldwide, Parkinson's disease prevalence and incidence studies show a marked geographical variation, ranging from 8.6 to 19 per 100,000 population per year. Because most Western studies quote prevalence rates of around 100-200 per 100,000 population. Studies in Australia, Korea and Singapore have shown incidences comparable to those reported in Western countries. Somewhat lower rates have been reported in Africa than in other geographic regions.

According to Dr. Dorsey et al. (2005) estimated that, in the most populous countries, the number of people with Parkinson's disease was close to 4.5 million in 2005 and that this figure would double by 2030. World Health Organisation projections also estimate an increase in the prevalence of Parkinson's disease due to the natural ageing process of the population.

In Chile, Parkinson's disease is "a relatively frequent entity in the elderly and has acquired interest as a public health problem since the 1990s, due to the increasing ageing of the population" (Sáenz de Pipaón and Larumbe, 2001, p. 61). This disease is considered one of the most important causes of disability in older adults, with a prevalence in the age range of 60 years and over as explained in the AUGE guide (2016), so that, based on INE estimates, it can be inferred that this disease has been increasing along with life expectancy, however, there are about 40,000 people with this disease in Chile according to the Ministry of Health (2013).

Currently, there are both pharmacological and non-pharmacological treatments for the disease, and it is here where occupational therapy is seen as a non-pharmacological solution that has as its central axis the promotion of autonomy and independence (Lear, 2015).

Parkinson's disease develops progressively, with consequences for the quality of life of people who suffer from it. It firstly affects people's performance and continues with alterations in participation in the different areas of occupation. The main objective of Occupational Therapy is to carry out a correct and exhaustive assessment of the practical problems that the person presents in their daily life, trying to remedy them in the best possible way, achieving the greatest possible independence and autonomy, maintaining their quality of life (Moruno and Romero, 2006).

The paucity of well-conducted studies in the area probably explains the limited use of occupational therapy intervention in the management and treatment of Parkinson's disease. At present, there is little evidence to adequately assess the effect of these interventions in people with Parkinson's disease, which is supported by several studies conducted between 1982 and 2004 which show that the provision of Occupational

Therapy in Parkinson's disease is very low, not exceeding 25%.

The focus of Occupational Therapy within public health is based on levels of care, which are health promotion and prevention, which within Parkinson's is focused on older adults prone to the disease and their caregivers. The treatment performed by the Occupational Therapist in people with Parkinson's Disease is the intervention through aspects that interfere with occupational performance, prolonging the time of independence within their activities of daily living respectively. On the other hand, it allows us to visualise the importance of complementary non-pharmacological therapies in this pathology, and how these can have a considerable influence on people's performance and, therefore, on their quality of life.

In the academic and rehabilitation field, this manual contributes to the current practice of Occupational Therapy, as it generates the need to reformulate prevention, diagnosis, treatment and prognosis, which are transformed into effective information strategies for future research. It also teaches how to rank the available evidence and thus learn to evaluate and categorise information. Finally, it allows the importance of placing the patient, his or her values and circumstances at the centre of medical and health care to become evident.

As discussed above, the above manifestations of Parkinson's disease have major repercussions, which incapacitate the person in many of their activities of daily living, and despite optimal medical or surgical treatment, they develop progressive disability. Both motor and non-motor symptoms and interaction with the environment can be very complex. This is why Occupational Therapy allows us to work under a holistic view, that is to say, we work with the person in unity of body, mind and spirit; giving the possibility of being able to carry out the intervention process together with the person.

The work of the Occupational Therapist is to give the person the opportunity to develop their life with maximum autonomy and satisfaction according to their objectives, personal motivations and the demands of the environment. Consequently, the Occupational Therapist becomes an active entity in terms of support and facilitation in order to maintain the usual level of activities carried out in the different areas of occupation for as long as possible. On the other hand, in more advanced stages, when it is no longer possible to maintain the usual level, the Occupational Therapist helps the person to change and adapt the way they relate to their physical and social environment in order to develop new roles and activities (Dixon, Duncan, Johnson, Kirkby, O'Connell and Taylor, 2017).

Worldwide, Parkinson's disease prevalence and incidence studies show a marked geographical variation, ranging from 8.6 to 19 per 100,000 population per year. Because most Western studies quote prevalence rates of around 100-200 per 100,000 population per year, the prevalence of Parkinson's disease is estimated to be between 8.6 and 19 per 100,000 population per year.
100,000 population. Studies in Australia, Korea and Singapore have shown incidences comparable to those reported in Western countries. Somewhat lower rates have been reported in Africa than in other geographical regions (Chaná, Alburquerque, Aránguiz, Baldwin, Benavides, de la Cerda, Curinao, Espinosa, Jeno, Juri, Kunstmann, Leyton, León, Rey, Sagua, Salazar, Tapia and Tapia, 2010).

In Chile, Parkinson's disease is "a relatively frequent entity in the elderly and has acquired interest as a public health problem since the 1990s, due to the increasing ageing of the population" (Sáenz de Pipaón and Larumbe, 2001, p. 61). This disease is considered one of the most important causes of disability in older adults, its prevalence being in the age range of 60 years and over as explained in the AUGE guide (2016), so based on INE estimates it can be inferred that this disease has been increasing along with life expectancy, however, there are about 40,000 people with this disease in Chile according to the Ministry of Health (2013).

A recent study published in "The Lancet Neurology", which included 954 prevalence studies, 34 incidence studies and 10 mortality risk studies in different countries around the world, concluded that in Chile during the period 1990 - 2016, deaths attributable to Parkinson's disease increased by

16.5% and prevalence by 19.9%, making it the Latin American country with the highest increase in the prevalence of Parkinson's disease, followed by Paraguay, El Salvador, among others.

Germán Cueto, neurologist at the Carlos Van Buren Hospital and professor at the University of Valparaíso analysed the complex scenario presented in this region due to the number of elderly people who suffer from Parkinson's disease, the specialist gave the results of his research where he explains that in Valparaíso 1.5% of the total number of older adults suffer from this disease and each year the figure is increasing by up to 300 new cases; it should be noted that this study also states that Valparaiso is one of the regions with a higher percentage of older adults reaching 15.7% which is equivalent to more than 270 thousand inhabitants, which is corroborated by the records of the National Service for the Elderly.

Parkinson's disease has made great advances over the years, both clinically and in terms of knowledge. One of the most important historical aspects of P.D. is the publication of James Parkinson in 1817, who described the clinical picture and semiology of the disease which is known today.

After James Parkinson's description, one of the most important events in the understanding of this pathology was the discovery of neuronal loss in the pars compacta of the substantia nigra, which was considered to be the characteristic lesion of P.E., a fact that still holds true today. Over the years, other milestones have marked an important development in the treatment of this disease, such as the description of cytoplasmic inclusion bodies of alpha-synuclein, described by Friederich Lewy, which received the name of Lewy bodies. Another of the findings was in 1919 where Konstantine Trétiakoff gave name to the substantia nigra, detailed its location and associated the loss of neurons in this area as part of the findings of P.E. (Arredondo, Zerón, Rodríguez and Cervantes, 2018).

There is literature and descriptions of the evolution of the treatment of P.E. dating back almost 3000 years, from Ayurvedic medicine through treatment with seeds containing high doses of Levodopa. The treatment of this disease has been a long evolutionary process. Dopamine was first synthesised in 1910 and then Levodopa in 1911, with Oleh Hornykiewicz in 1979 being the first to propose the use of Levodopa for the treatment of the disease. From this point on, there were many advances in pharmacological treatment, the efficacy of Levodopa became evident, but the long-term side effects were also known. However, it was introduced in conjunction with dopamine inhibitors, which is one of the most widely used drugs today. Subsequently, dopamine agonists were initially approved in the 1970s and 1980s, considered a major breakthrough in the pharmacological treatment of this disease (Arredondo et al., 2018).

On the other hand, the last of the important findings in the treatment of this pathology is surgical intervention, which has been used since 1908, but it was not until 1987 that the birth of deep brain stimulation was established, a surgical technique that has evolved over the years and together with technology, and which today is used in the treatment of the disease.
E.P. (Arredondo et al., 2018).

Parkinson's disease has been studied for approximately 200 years, with the aim of understanding and identifying the aetiology, pathophysiology and developing treatments to alleviate the symptoms, modify the progression and evolution of the disease and, finally, to reach a cure that helps to improve the quality of life of people suffering from this disease (Arredondo et al., 2018).

For many years, the concept of health has been understood as the absence of a disease and its symptomatology without considering the consequences that these entail in people's lives, however, it has become obsolete since, at present, this concept is linked to the well-being of people and their full participation in the contexts in which they work. This concept has evolved over the years in the field of disability and after Chile started using the International Classification of Functioning, Disability and Health (ICF) there was a great positive impact on rehabilitation teams (Chaná et al., 2010).

Occupational therapy has been recognised as a fundamental part of the rehabilitation process for people with PD, however, it has been questioned in the areas of strategy, task, effectiveness and cost, due to factors such as the scarcity of controlled, validated studies or inadequate methods used in treatment. Despite this, there is evidence of the importance of rehabilitation in the functional recovery of people with PD, both in the reduction of symptomatology and in daily activities, motor performance and aspects of personal confidence (Chaná et al. 2010).

The basic objectives for every treatment and rehabilitation of people suffering from the disease is to achieve maximum independence in activities of daily living. Occupational therapy is fundamentally aimed at restoring compromised muscles and joints, improving coordination of movements, increasing work tolerance time, stimulating cognitive activity and improving overall physical conditions (Hernández, 2015).

In recent years, the rehabilitation of Parkinson's disease has been a topic of interest for many specialists, as disability is present at all stages of the disease, thus affecting the quality of life of the person. Even in the early stages of the disease, it can lead to dependence in activities of daily living such as hygiene, dressing, eating and other activities (Hernández et al., 2015).

If a large part of occupational therapy interventions have been "evidence-based", what is the contribution of scientific evidence to current clinical practice in Parkinson's disease? (Rodriguez, 2009).

- Rethink how to turn the need for information into questions of prevention, diagnosis, treatment and prognosis, which must be transformed into strategies and effective information seeking.
- Generate the need to optimise bibliographic search strategies in the world of information as wide-ranging as that found on the internet, scientific journals, among others.
- Generate critical reading strategies, using published tools that

simplify the task of assessing scientific information.

- Enable the generation of systematic reviews and the development of meta-analyses that are essential for decision-making in medical practice.

- It allows you to rank the available evidence and thus learn to assess and categorise the available information.

- To be able to generate the creation of large databases, in which groups of experts select and analyse scientific studies from the most important journals.

- Generate the need to democratise and disseminate scientific information more efficiently and make some important journals open access.

- The combination of "best evidence" and clinical expertise allows a better quality of care to be offered to patients from a medical technical point of view.

- In the philosophy of EBM, the patient, his or her values, preferences and circumstances are placed as the most important aspect of the medical act and health care, making it clear that patients' values and preferences do not always match our own, so it is of utmost importance to always take this into account.

- It has changed the way decisions are made in the treatment of Parkinson's disease, from the traditionally vertical way, with little or no patient participation in the care of their health, to a horizontal way of making decisions. The process begins with the formulation of a clinical problem related to the patient, the evaluation of their clinical condition, their circumstances and generates a research question, bibliographic sources are consulted, the information obtained is integrated with clinical experience and finally it is combined with the values and preferences of the patient, in order to solve the problem presented.

In conclusion, in decision making in any rehabilitation treatment in therapy as well as in other disciplines, evidence alone is never enough, as adequate diagnosis, careful risk/benefit assessment, cost assessment and patient values and preferences are required.

Parkinson's disease is a neurodegenerative disorder with a chronic and irreversible course, which causes progressive disability in the patient and has no known cause (Martínez, 2010). The fundamental lesion lies in the compact part of the substantia nigra (SN), which is part of the basal ganglia (GB). Despite the above, the cause is probably multifactorial, with the main aetiological factors being genetic and environmental in nature (Guía Minsal Enfermedad de Parkinson, 2010).

The aforementioned manifestations have a significant impact and incapacitate the patient in many of their daily activities, resulting in a significant loss of self-esteem as well as in the expression of feelings of worthlessness and hopelessness.

On the other hand, Durante (2010) argues that Parkinson's disease is known to be slow and degenerative in origin, resulting in the loss of neurons in the substantia nigra and other basal ganglia, leading to a decrease in the neurotransmitter dopamine, which is involved in the regulation of various functions, specifically motor behaviour. He also adds that it is characterised by the presence of rigidity, mainly in the arms, legs and neck, tremor at rest, bradykinesia and altered postural reflexes.

Parkinson's disease is one of the oldest chronic degenerative disorders on record. In India it was known as kampavata and Galen gave it the name "paralysis agitans".

However, it was the British physician James Parkinson who, on the basis of his own clinical observations of six patients, published in 1817 an essay with the first systematic and comprehensive description of paralysis agitans, in which for the first time details of the disease were specifically recorded from the observation of the participants. At that time it became known that tremor, bradykinesia and postural instability are the most important signs of this entity. Parkinson stated that this was an "involuntary trembling movement... in parts which are not in activity" and noted the "propensity to flex the trunk forward" (Parkinson, 1817). In describing the natural history of the disease it was revealed that the onset of the disease was slowly progressive, starting unilaterally and within a short time involving the contralateral side of the body, with subsequent involvement of the upright walking position and development of antepulsion of gait. He mentioned that as time progressed, the patient felt that movements lost precision and were performed with great difficulty. Falls became more noticeable due to the inability to easily raise the legs and speech became intelligible, requiring the constant presence of a caregiver. Perhaps one of his most significant considerations today was the description of some non-motor symptoms of the disease, for example, sleep disturbances, constipation, sialorrhoea and sphincter disturbances (Arredondo, Zerón, Rodríguez and Cervantes, 2017).

The degenerative picture involved in Parkinson's disease affects different areas of the central nervous system, whose symptoms appear due to a decrease in dopamine-producing cells, located in the substantia nigra pars compacta of the basal nuclei, and the presence of Lewys bodies in neurons. Lewys bodies are intracytoplasmic inclusions that are concentrated in neurons throughout the central nervous system (De la Vega and Zambrano, 2009), mainly in the basal nuclei, substantia nigra, locus coeruleus, dorsal motor nucleus of the vagus and Meynert's nucleus, and their presence may be necessary for the diagnosis of Parkinson's disease, but has also been seen in other degenerative diseases.

Also, pale bodies, which are other inclusions located in the neuronal bodies in this disease, are observed, which could be the precursors of Lewys bodies (Micheli, 2002). As discussed above, the cause of this degeneration is unknown, but the mechanisms of neuronal death are similar to other conditions, such as Alzheimer's disease. These mechanisms include oxidative stress, excitotoxicity, inflammation and apoptosis (Yáñez, 2011).

Cell apoptosis is a programmed cell death or destruction pathway triggered by the organism itself, in order to control its development and growth, which is triggered by genetically controlled cell signals. Apoptosis is therefore considered as a physiological natural death, resulting in a mechanism of elimination of unwanted, damaged or unknown cells and playing a protective role against possible diseases (Rommy von Bernhardi, 2004).

Oxidative stress or redox imbalance can be defined as a state in which the production of free radicals and the damage they can generate exceed the capacity of cells to eliminate reactive species and promote the efficient recovery of their most important molecules (DNA, proteins and lipids). The relationship of this phenomenon with the neurodegenerative processes occurring in Parkinson's disease may be associated with the characteristics of the human brain, an organ that has high levels of easily peroxidised fatty acids, consumes 20% of the oxygen incorporated in the bloodstream, and is not specifically enriched in antioxidant enzymes (Almaguer, 2006).

According to Gómez, Roldan, Morales, Pérez and Torner (2012) the pathological feature of Parkinson's disease is "the pronounced loss of dopamine-producing neurons located in the substantia nigra pars compacta (SNpc); these cells normally release dopamine at their axon terminals in the striatum and are part of the pyramidal system of motor regulation" (p.1). Further mentioning that, these pathogenic mechanisms that deteriorate the neurons of the substantia nigra would lead to neuronal death, a process in which dopamine-dependent oxidative stress is involved. This oxidative stress is a harmful condition produced by the deficient elimination of reactive oxygen species that affect dopaminergic neurons.

Gómez et al. (2012) report that dopaminergic cells under normal Ph conditions are exposed to oxidative stress by dopamine metabolism itself (auto-oxidation), which produces molecules that act as endogenous neurotoxins (dopamine quinone, superoxide radicals and hydrogen peroxide). In addition, they can be catalysed by monoamine oxidase (MAO), which leads to reactions that also produce hydrogen peroxide. This hydrogen peroxide alone is not capable of damaging the neuron, however, it can induce cytotoxicity by forming hydroxyl free radicals due to an iron-catalysed reaction. On the other hand, with respect to the above, the authors indicate that the reactive oxygen species produced during dopamine metabolism caused some alterations in the functions of DNA proteins and neuronal lipids, which would result in a modification of the ionic permeability of the membrane, affecting the electrical properties and, therefore, increasing toxicity.

Gómez et al. (2012) also mention that it is essential for dopamine to be harmless to the neuron, which takes place when it is stored rapidly within the synaptic vesicles, thanks to the low pH and absence of monoamine oxidase (MAO); this being the main mechanism by which neurons in the substantia nigra protect themselves from the damaging effects of dopamine oxidation. Normally, the reactive species are eliminated by intracellular antioxidant systems, however, according to the authors, these were damaged due to a normal ageing process or some pathological alteration. Finally, the authors report that the cells of the substantia nigra are at a high level of oxidative stress in Parkinson's disease.

Although this is the neurophysiological process that justifies the decrease in dopaminergic producing cells. There is a chain of pathophysiological processes that trigger the characteristic symptomatology of P.E. that are also closely related to neuroanatomical structures. The basal ganglia are a group of subcortical nuclei that control voluntary movements including: the striatum (putamen and caudate), globus pallidus, subthalamic nucleus and substantia nigra. The basal ganglia have no direct connections to the descending tracts of the medulla, but form nerve circuits of four types with the motor cortex: motor, oculomotor, promoter and limbic. These different circuits appear to control movements with varying levels of complexity and in different anatomical areas. The main neurotransmitters are glutamate and gamma-amino butyric acid (GABA). The circuits contain direct (excitatory) and indirect (inhibitory) pathways. The lack of inhibition of populations of neurons in the motor cortex appears to allow certain physical movements of P.E. to occur

(Martinez, Gasca, Sanchez, & Obeso, 2016).

Due to the loss of dopaminergic stimulation there is a potentiation of the so-called indirect pathway over the direct or "facilitatory" pathway of movement. The lack of dopamine results in hyperactivity (increased discharge rate) of the NST and the Gpi/SNr complex and, therefore, thalamo-cortical inhibition (Martínez et al., 2016).

The lack of dopamine results in a tendency of neurons in the GBs to discharge in an oscillatory manner instead of the physiological tonic activation. Due to the multiple interconnections between the GBs and their interconnections with the thalamus and cortex, this pathological discharge pattern is synchronised throughout the system, unlike what happens under normal physiological conditions in which the neuronal discharge pattern is functionally specific for each nucleus (Martínez et al., 2016).

The neuroanatomical component responsible for the main clinical manifestations in P.E. is the dysfunction of the Basal Ganglia system, due to the decrease of dopamine, which is its main modulator as mentioned above.

The onset of clinical manifestations is predominantly asymmetric and insidious in onset. The preclinical latency period has been estimated at five to ten years, although it may be variable depending on the aetiology. Degenerative damage to multiple neural systems results in complex biochemical and pathophysiological alterations that may explain the clinical heterogeneity of PD. Cardinal manifestations or signs within Parkinson's disease include low frequency resting tremor, muscle rigidity, slowness, poor movement and impaired postural recovery reflexes (Michelli, 2006).

Motor symptoms

As mentioned above, rigidity, bradykinesia, resting tremor and impaired postural reflexes are the four main motor symptoms of P.E.

Stiffness is defined as increased resistance to passive mobilisation of a joint segment, i.e. when attempting to flex or extend a joint, resistance to passive mobilisation is evident. In Parkinsonian syndromes it affects both flexor and extensor muscles, although more so the flexors. It usually varies in intensity during passive movement, giving rise to the so-called "cogwheel". In advanced stages the resistance to passive movement is uniform and is then referred to as "lead bar" rigidity. The rigidity differs from the increased tone of pyramidal neurological diseases, because when initial resistance is applied, it gives way abruptly at some point in the movement, giving rise to the Razor phenomenon (Micheli, 2002). On the other hand, Zarranz (2013) indicates that rigidity would be the product of hyperactivity produced in the subthalamic nucleus, which would excite the internal globus pallidus. In addition, he mentions that stereotaxic lesions could reduce rigidity and be used in the treatment of Parkinson's disease.

Tremor is the most characteristic sign, with a prevalence of 70% to 80% of patients with P.E. It is a low frequency tremor (4 to 6 Hz), associated with alternating contractions of antagonistic muscles. It develops progressively and asymmetrically, initially affecting one of the four limbs or body segments such as the jaw, tongue, head, among others, and then expands and ends contralaterally (Micheli, 2002). This sign appears during rest; it is an involuntary movement. It is rhythmic and generally decreases when performing a movement of the structure that manifests a problem; it may disappear when sleeping or when adopting a posture; it may also increase when faced with sudden changes in emotions.

According to Micheli (2006), the pathophysiology of resting tremor is unknown, however, it is likely to originate in thalamic generators. The author states that "peripheral afferents may modulate tremor in P.E., but it persists after deafferentation, demonstrating that, despite the modulation exerted by afferents, central activity is critical for tremor development" (p.174-175). It is currently unknown which cerebellar mechanism is involved in Parkinson's disease, and it is not known why the thalamic generator is activated, but it is thought that inhibitory dysfunction in the internal globus pallidus may trigger and activate this mechanism (Micheli, 2006).

Bradykinesia is an extrapyramidal disorder characterised by a slowing of movements. The term is used to refer to slowness of movement, i.e. the poverty of voluntary movements due to a failure of initiation. The movements of these patients are executed slowly despite the correct motor strategy. Clinically it is manifested by a poverty in all types of movement, loss of automatic movements, delay in initiating a movement and reduction of the amplitude of voluntary movements; it can culminate in complete immobility. On the other hand, according to Zarranz (2013), bradykinesia would be associated with a decrease in activity in the supplementary motor area and the prefrontal and dorsolateral cortex.

In Parkinson's disease, there are episodes called freezing, a phenomenon related to the difficulty in initiating voluntary movements that occur when attempting to turn or start walking. In relation to bradykinesia, there is also postural instability in patients, presenting an important problem in the postural reflexes that allow a rapid change in muscle tone to maintain posture. It is the main cause of falls and loss of autonomy (Micheli, 2002). The pathophysiology of this clinical sign is poorly understood, this could be related to an abnormal execution of higher motor programmes, possibly in the supplementary motor cortex (Micheli, 2006).

Finally, postural instability. Patients with Parkinson's disease have impaired postural fixation, balance and uprighting, especially in advanced stages of the disease. They often adopt a flexed posture of the head and trunk and are unable to make postural adjustments to lean, support themselves or straighten up. They also have a tendency to move with short, rapid steps in an uncontrolled manner, performing a so-called festinating gait.

According to Micheli (2006), the pathophysiology related to postural instability is not directly related to a failure in the use of sensory information or a prolonged latency of the postural response, but rather to inflexible and uncoordinated postural movement patterns, which are inefficient for the changing conditions of the environment. The main cause could be due to an overactivity of certain archaic long latency reflexes, different from transcortical stretch reflexes.

Non-motor symptoms

The implication of non-motor symptoms (NMS) lies in the impact on the quality of life of patients, becoming the cause of hospitalisations of subjects. These symptoms may be present in the early stages of the disease, even ten years before the onset of motor symptoms, and become more evident as P.E. progresses (Chaudhuri and Schapira, 2009).

Studies have shown that MNS preceding the motor signs of P.E. correlate closely with the progression of Lewy's pathology in this disease, as deposits of these are found in the olfactory bulb. Projections from the substantia nigra mediate non-motor symptoms such as cognition, sleep and pain (Aguilera, Pacheco, Núñez and Colina, 2017).

The main non-motor symptoms are, among others:

Psychiatric symptoms: Comprising cognitive and neuropsychiatric symptoms (Chaudhuri and Schapira, 2009; Macias, 2006; Parrao, Cuevas, Claverías, Kunstmann and Tapia, 2005; Stella, Bucken, Gobbi, and Sant'Ana, 2007), these are:
- Depression: This is an important and common symptom, affecting 40-45% of patients. Depression has been observed as a predecessor to motor symptoms and as an enabler of Parkinson's disease persistence.
- Apathy: This is a specific symptom of P.E. that may or may not be accompanied by depression and/or anxiety. It is defined as a lack of interest and motivation, accompanied by reduced thought content and affective flattening. Anxiety: Frequent, with a prevalence of 20-38%, especially in the early stages of the disease. It manifests as general restlessness, agitation, chronic anxiety, phobic disorders and panic attacks.

- Dementia: It is progressive and is characterised by a gradual loss of memory and intellectual capacity, as well as loss of judgement and personality changes. Estimated prevalence is between 20-40%.
- Specific cognitive impairment: This is a common symptom in advanced P.E., however, it can be found in early stages presenting as an alteration in frontal executive function. Neuropsychological impairments in memory, cognitive processing speed, visuospatial functions and frontal functions have been described.

Sleep disorders

Dopamine plays a complex role in the sleep-wake cycle. These disorders tend to worsen over time and occur in 60-98% of subjects (Chaudhuri and Schapira, 2009). Sleep disorders correlate with P.E. severity, Levodopa dose, bradykinesia and rigidity.

- Insomnia: Difficulty falling asleep and the inability to maintain sleep are common in P.E.
- Restless legs syndrome and periodic leg movements: This is understood as the imperious need to move the legs,

    They may be preceded by paraesthesias or dysesthesias and are predominantly nocturnal. Prevalence is 68%.
- REM sleep disorder: Present in up to 47% of P.E. patients, it correlates with the severity and duration of the disease. It consists of aggressive behaviour associated with nightmares or vivid dreams occurring in REM sleep, which is characterised by expected muscle atonia.
- Daytime sleepiness: This is defined as a feeling of constant sleepiness, with peak daytime sleepiness. It is present in about 50% of subjects with P.E. and correlates with age, severity and duration of the disease.

Sensory/sensory symptoms (Chaudhuri and Schapira, 2009):

- Pain: Dopamine modulates pain at various levels of the nervous system. Some authors suggest that pain is based on dysfunction of dopamine-dependent autonomic centres that regulate autonomic functions and pain inhibition.
- Visual dysfunction: Colour and contrast discrimination are affected in this field. Diplopia, blurred vision and difficulty in reading have also been reported. It may affect approximately 78% of P.E. subjects.
- Hyposmia: Affects 90%. It is the early loss of smell and can occur years before the development of the disease, as well as correlating with the progression of the disease.
- Rhinorrhoea: This is caused by a decrease in sympathetic tone in the nasal mucosa, so that parasympathetic innervation prevails,

stimulating nasal secretion.

In the development of this pathology, six stages can be distinguished, where the symptomatology becomes more severe over the years. These stages are based on the Hoehn and Yahr Scale for assessing the progression and severity of Parkinson's disease (Guía Minsal Enfermedad de Parkinson, 2010).

- Stage 0: No signs of disease.
- Stage 1: Unilateral disease.
- Stage 2: Bilateral disease, without balance disturbance.
- Stage 3: Mild to moderate bilateral disease with postural instability; physically independent.
- Stage 4: Severe disability, still able to walk or stand unaided.
- Stage 5: Remains wheelchair-bound or bedridden if unaided.

According to Martínez et al. (2016), as Parkinson's disease progresses and advances, the motor manifestations that were previously present in one side of the body extend to affect the contralateral side, maintaining a degree of asymmetry in its evolution. As the deterioration progresses, axial manifestations appear, affecting alterations in postural reflexes, gait magnetisation, hypophonia, dysarthria and dysphagia, which are highly disabling. The authors Martínez et al. (2016) report that studies have shown that after
20 years of disease progression, approximately 87% of people suffer from falls and 81% from gait magnetisation, being the main problems of P.E. In advanced stages because the body no longer responds as efficiently to dopaminergic treatment.

On the other hand, Martínez et al. (2016) report that in recent years, non-motor symptoms or manifestations have taken on great relevance in the development of this disease, due to its high prevalence and negative impact on the quality of life of people suffering from this disease. Martínez et al. (2016) state that "despite their relevance, non-motor symptoms in P.E. are often little known, probably because medical consultation focuses primarily on motor manifestations" (p.4).

According to the authors Castro and Buriticá (2014), the diagnosis of Parkinson's disease is based on clinical suspicion, as there are no specific chemical or radiological markers to establish it. Martínez et al. (2016) mention that for a definitive diagnosis to be made, it is necessary to confirm neuropathological findings such as neuronal loss of the SNc and the presence of Lewy bodies and neurites, which can only be carried out when the person has died.

Currently the most commonly used criteria are from the UKPDSBB (United Kingdom Parkinson's Disease Society Brain Bank), which are considered to have a diagnostic certainty of 90% (Castro and Buriticá, 2014).

Step 1: Diagnosis of Parkinsonian Syndrome
●Bradicinesia (slow initiation of voluntary movement with progressive reduction in speed and amplitude of repetitive actions).   ●At least one of the following: -Muscle rigidity   -Resting tremor of 4-6 Hz;   -Postural instability not caused by visual, vestibular, cerebellar or proprioceptive compromise.
Step 2: Exclusion criteria for P.E.

History of repeated strokes or stepwise progression of parkinsonian signs.
• History   of repeated head trauma.
• History   of encephalitis.
•   Oculogyric crises   .
•Neuroleptic treatment   at symptom onset.
•More than   one affected relative.
•Sustained transmission.
Unilateral symptoms   after 3 years of evolution.
•   Supranuclear gaze palsy.
•   Cerebellar signs.
•Early and severe autonomous engagement.
•   Early dementia   with memory, language and praxis disorders.
•   Babinski's sign.
• Presence   of brain tumour or communicating hydrocephalus on CT scan.
Lack of response to adequate doses of Levodopa (if malabsorption is excluded).
•Exposure   to MPTP toxin.

Step 3: Criteria supporting the diagnosis of P.E.

Three or more are required for a definitive diagnosis of P.E.).
•   Unilateral start.
•   Resting tremor.
•Progressive frame   .
Persistent asymmetry   that involves more of the side on which it started.
•Excellent   response (70-100%) to Levodopa.
•Levodopa-induced severe chorea.
•Levodopa response   of 5 years or more.
•Clinical course   of 10 years or more.

Table 1: UK Parkinson's Disease Society Brain Bank clinical criteria (Castro and Buritica, 2014).

Martínez et al. (2016) state that a detailed anamnesis and neurological examination are essential to reach a clinical diagnosis. During the anamnesis, the slowly progressive course of the cardinal motor symptoms should be highlighted, as well as their distribution, which is typically asymmetrical. On the other hand, the authors indicate that it is essential to question the person about their medication, since there are several drugs that have a dopaminergic blocking action that can induce pharmacological parkinsonism. With regard to the neurological examination, the main motor manifestations of P.S. such as tremor at rest, rigidity and bradykinesia should be observed, in addition to ruling out atypical signs suggestive of other causes of parkinsonism such as: supranuclear gaze palsy, cerebellar or balance disorders, clinically significant cognitive deficits of early onset, cortical signs such as motor apraxia or alterations in cortical sensitivity and autonomic dysfunction. Finally, the authors mention that another way to support the diagnosis is through a "therapeutic trial" with Levodopa, as P.E. responds effectively to the use of this drug, whereas in secondary and atypical parkinsonisms, the response is limited.

Pharmacological treatment in Parkinson's disease:

Although Parkinson's disease has been constantly studied for years, to this day there are no satisfactory treatment results.

One of the ways to intervene is through pharmacological treatment. The dopamine precursor Levodopa or L-Dopa, as indicated by Hurtado, Cárdenas, Cárdenas and León (2016), improves the quality of life of people by alleviating the motor symptoms that they present, however, over time it loses its effectiveness, However, over time it loses its effectiveness, producing long-term side effects such as dyskinesias, which affect the activities of daily living of people with Parkinson's disease, which is why it is recommended to start treatment with dopamine agonists, which delay the onset of motor complications.

According to the Minsal Guide for Parkinson's Disease (2010),

Levodopa is the most effective drug for the treatment of PD, improving symptoms such as rigidity, bradykinesia, gait disturbances, hypomimia and micrographia, as well as having an effect on tremor, but to a lesser extent. Levodopa is a drug that is absorbed in the gastrointestinal tract and there it crosses the blood-brain barrier and is converted to dopamine by the action of the enzyme L-amino acid aromatic decarboxylase (LAAD). Current Levodopa preparations have an added decarboxylase inhibitor (carbidopa or benserazide), these do not cross the blood-brain barrier, inhibiting conversion at the peripheral, but not the central level, in order to minimise systemic side effects and reduce the daily requirement of this drug. Finally, Levodopa treatment has a rapid response, so if people do not improve their symptoms, it may not be P.S.

On the other hand, dopaminergic agonists, according to Figueira (2012), delay the onset of motor complications in the treatment of Parkinson's disease. However, some of these can cause serious side effects such as hypotension, gastrointestinal disorders, retroperitoneal fibrosis, hallucinations, psychosis, pleuropulmonary complications, dizziness, drowsiness, among others. However, pramipexole, which is a dopamine agonist that has been evaluated in the treatment of people with early and advanced Parkinson's disease, has demonstrated low side effects and has been well tolerated by people.

Dopamine agonists such as pramipexole are not as effective in treating the symptoms of Parkinson's disease compared to Levodopa which remains the best drug for symptomatic treatment, however, it has greater durability, being useful in the treatment in the early stages and complementary in the advanced stages together with L-dopa concluding that it delays the onset of motor complications such as dyskinesias compared to people who take an initial treatment with Levodopa (Figueira, 2012).

After a certain number of years, pharmacological treatment begins to diminish in effectiveness and the symptoms of the disease reappear, accompanied by the side effects of the drugs. This is where deep brain stimulation (DBS) comes in, a surgical treatment which focuses on electrical stimuli directed towards cortical or subcortical areas.

According to Rodríguez, Cervantes and Arellano (2014), this technique is of great help in the treatment of people who present motor alterations or complications, including dyskinesias resulting from Levodopa treatment, helping to improve performance in activities of daily living. De la Peña, Fernández, Parra and Martínez (2016) point out that "deep brain stimulation (DBS) is a safe and effective surgical technique that has been shown to improve the quality of life of patients with P.E., both in motor symptoms and neuropsychological manifestations".

Non-pharmacological treatment in Parkinson's disease.
While it is true that Parkinson's disease has no cure as such, what is expected with pharmacological and non-pharmacological treatments is to slow down the deterioration that exists in the person over the years. According to the Minsal Guide for Parkinson's Disease (2010), there are different professionals who play a fundamental role in the process of involution of the disease.

One of them is Kinesthetic rehabilitation, whose main objective is to maintain the quality of life of those suffering from the disease, helping to improve mobility, balance, coordination and maintain the person's autonomy for a longer period of time.

In addition, there must be education together with the family, caregivers and the community in general, so that they play an active role in the rehabilitation process (Guía Minsal Enfermedad de Parkinson, 2010).

INITIAL PHASE	Preventing and treating postural instability early assessment and identification of problems related to movement disorders.
	Encourage participation in programmes designed to improve physical fitness (cardiovascular, musculoskeletal and neuromuscular).
	Prevent postural deficiencies, gait and transfer deficiencies.
	Use movement strategies throughout the course of the disease.
	Educating patients, families and carers.
	To assess pharmacological efficacy on motor performance.
PHASE OF	Assess the functional capacity of the person.

Table 2:

MAINTENANCE	Treating musculoskeletal deterioration.
	Re-educate walking, falls and transfers.
	Assess the environment in which the person develops, in order to achieve good training within the home and community.
	Educate family members and caregivers to encourage movement and good patient management.
ADVANCED OR LATE STAGE	Education and counselling in the proper management of the person's mobility and positioning.
	Avoid the risk of falls.
	Establish an exercise regimen, taking into account age, cognitive impairment and the multiple disorders that may have triggered the disease in the person.

Description of kinesthetic recommendations in the treatment of people with Parkinson's disease according to their stage of evolution, Guía Minsal Enfermedad de Parkinson (2010). p.28.

On the other hand, Phonoaudiology is defined as a scientific discipline, which is in charge of evaluating, diagnosing, intervening and rehabilitating people who suffer from a symptom frequently observed in early stages called dysphonia. This is due to the loss of dopaminergic input in the striatum and consequently the dysregulation of the basal ganglia, producing a motor deficit that negatively affects the three subsystems related to the motor control of speech: respiratory, phonatory and articulatory (Delgado and Izquierdo, 2016).

As they present progressive alterations in their speech, swallowing and language, affecting their general state and quality of life, the care of the children and adolescents is essential.
implemented according to the following scheme, always taking into consideration the stages of the disease in which the person is:

INITIAL PHASE	Objective: Prevention procedures: Initial assessment, treatment, education and reassessment. Frequency: 5 sessions per year are recommended.
ADVANCED STAGE	Objective: Rehabilitation Procedures: Initial assessment, treatment, reassessment. Frequency: 10 sessions per year are recommended.
PROSTRATION PHASE	Objective: Rehabilitation Procedures: Initial assessment, treatment, reassessment. Frequency: 10 sessions per year are recommended.

Table 3: Description of objectives, procedures and frequency of sessions to be considered according to phonoaudiology. Guía Minsal Enfermedad de Parkinson (2010). p.29.

As mentioned in the Guía Minsal Enfermedad de Parkinson (2010):

"Psychological support aims at a "good acceptance of the disease", with a general orientation towards behavioural, mainly emotional, management. Aspects such as: training in guidelines for coping with depression, distress, anxiety, apathy, social inhibition, fear of the future, frustration, should be the focus of such support. Along with this, it is necessary to give help to the patient's environment: family and caregivers" (p.30).

It is recommended, according to the stages of the disease:

INITIAL PHASE	six sessions: one assessment session and five sessions of individual psychotherapy. 4 sessions of group psychotherapy (8 to 12 patients).
ADVANCED STAGE	6 sessions of individual psychotherapy. 4 sessions of psychosocial intervention (8 to 12 patients), Family members and/or carers).
PROSTRATION PHASE	six sessions of individual psychotherapy. 4 sessions psychosocial intervention (8 to 12 to family members and/or carers).

Table 4: Description of sessions to be considered according to psychological support. Guía Minsal enfermedad de Parkinson (2010). p.30.

Occupational Therapy Intervention in Parkinson's Disease.

Polonio (2015), mention that Parkinson's Disease is one of the most frequent neurodegenerative disorders in Occupational Therapy services, due to the fact that it is a chronic, progressive and disabling disease that produces, to a greater or lesser extent, a decrease in the quality of life of the person suffering from it and those living with it. It is also the second most frequent degenerative neuropathology in our environment, after Alzheimer's disease (Polonio, 2015).

One of the best known definitions of Occupational Therapy (OT) is from the American Occupational Therapy Association (AOTA, 2014), which states that it is "The therapeutic use of activities of daily living (occupations) with individuals or groups for the purpose of enhancing or enabling participation in roles, habits, and routines in the home, school, workplace, community, and other settings (AOTA, 2014, p. 1).

The main aim of Occupational Therapy is to ensure that the person affected is as independent and autonomous as possible, in order to improve and/or maintain their quality of life. With the person suffering from Parkinson's disease, Occupational Therapy performs very specific functions that are defined by the pathology itself, the state and evolution of the disease in each subject and the personal circumstances of each individual.

The focus of Occupational Therapy within public health is based on levels of care, which are health promotion and prevention, which within Parkinson's is focused on older adults prone to the disease and their caregivers. The Occupational Therapist's treatment of people with Parkinson's Disease is the intervention through aspects that interfere with occupational performance, prolonging the time of independence within their activities of daily living respectively.

Occupational performance is the realisation of the selected occupation, resulting from the interaction between the client, the context, the environment and the activity or occupation (AOTA, 2014).

According to the Canadian Occupational Therapy Association, occupational performance is defined as: "The connection between the person, the environment in which they live and the occupation they perform, being a dynamic interaction between the person, the environment and the occupation" (Law, Polatajko, Baptiste and Townsend, 1997, p. 2).

Occupational performance can be described as "a dynamic relationship between an occupational form, a person with a unique developmental structure, and a person with a unique developmental structure".

with subjective purposes and meanings, an environment in which he or she operates and the occupation he or she performs within the same context (Nelson and Thomas, 2003).

According to the Occupational Therapy intervention in Parkinson's disease, the main functions are to perform a comprehensive assessment of the state in which the person is, their environment and how this influences the different areas of performance, specifically in those activities that require a more complex cognitive component and require a more personal autonomy such as activities of daily living. According to AOTA (2010), activities of daily living are defined as activities that are oriented towards caring for one's own body, which are fundamental for living in a social world, allowing for survival and well-being.

The main objective of Occupational Therapy during non-pharmacological treatment is to enable people to participate in activities of daily living. While it is a complex process based on the cooperative interaction between the professional, the multidisciplinary team and the person, immersed in the context of intervention. The intervention, as determined by the Hoehn and Yahr scale, is then outlined.

INITIAL STAGE (H & Y: 0 to 2)	-To carry out a diagnosis of occupational participation: with an emphasis on prevention.
	-Carry out a diagnosis of the support networks, using the Network Map.
	-Assessing the family situation: emphasising prevention of caregiver overload.
	-Prevention of social isolation. -Support in the bereavement phase of the illness.
	- Encouragement of participation in meaningful activities, to maintain a balanced and satisfying life routine. -Modality of care: individual and group care. family members.
INTERMEDIATE STAGE (H&Y 2, and 3)	Identification of problems in activities of daily living, productivity and leisure time.
	Rehabilitation towards maintaining occupational performance in meaningful activities.
	Stimulation of motor, processing, and communication and interaction skills.

Identification of the new condition of the person's performance, favouring autonomy and independence.
Falls prevention: Assessment and modification of the contexts in which the person performs.
Orthotics and fittings
Evidence of elements of caregiver overload.
Restructuring of life routines in favour of the maintenance of the person and his/her family members in activities of interest, avoiding the loss of participation in social and community instances of all family members.
Maintenance of support networks. Assess performance issues in social and work contexts for physical and social intervention.
Facilitating the generation of self-help groups. Emphasis on processes in a community context.
Modality of care: Individual and family sessions. Home and community visits. Intervention from a more functionalist perspective, performance, independence and autonomy

ADVANCED STAGE (H&Y: 4 to 5)	Emphasis of the intervention on the caregiver, for the management of the affected person in favour of the quality of life of the family group.
	Assessment of the person's occupational performance (used suggested guideline that can be answered by the caregiver).
	Determination of critical areas.
	Assessment of caregiver overload (Zarit).
	Training of assistance in activities of daily living, favouring as much independence as possible (collaboration, choice in certain steps of the task).
	Prevention of injuries due to caregiver overload, postural education, environmental management, use of bars, transfer elements, adaptations in bathrooms, bedrooms, etc.
	Structuring of life routines, providing leisure and free time for the caregiver. Use of family and community support networks.

Table 5: Description of sessions to be considered according to psychological support. Guía Minsal enfermedad de Parkinson (2010). p.30 - 31.

According to the authors Gómez, Matilla and Fernández (2020),

Parkinson's disease is neurodegenerative, therefore, occupational therapy intervention should be based on prevention and maintenance work.

On the other hand, the educational process that takes place is fundamental for the health of people suffering from this disease, as well as for family members and caregivers, in order to achieve a more effective and successful treatment.

Before starting treatment, an assessment must be made, which is carried out through the use of various standardised guidelines and through clinical observation. In addition, Gómez et al. (2020) point out that, in order to explain the treatment more effectively, it has been divided into five phases according to the level of severity of the person. On the other hand, the Minsal Guide for Parkinson's Disease (2010), organises the Occupational Therapy intervention in three moments based on the Hoehn and Yahr scale according to the progression of the disease which was mentioned above.

As mentioned by the authors Gómez et al. (2020), the intervention is divided into five phases which indicate the following:

- Phase I: Regarding this phase, the authors indicate that the intervention will be mainly aimed at maintaining and slowing down cognitive and motor deterioration, in order to maintain the person's independence for as long as possible. This phase focuses on certain aspects such as maintaining postural alignment, balance, muscle tone and muscle group training to prevent tendon retractions and joint limitations. In addition, this phase prioritises gait training and maintenance of waist dissociation, which helps in the prevention of future falls. Other aspects to work on are the maintenance of hand functionality, breathing and relaxation exercises and finally, a very important aspect is health education, i.e. advising the person on compensatory aids, explaining and making them aware of the importance of physical activity and the management of non-motor symptoms.

-   Phase II: The authors mention that, in this phase, the person is already bilaterally affected, therefore, when the same affectation is present in the other hemibody, all the work mentioned in phase I will be maintained. In addition, compensatory strategies and energy conservation techniques are added.

-   Phase III: Regarding this phase, the authors mention that work will be done in the ON phase if present (in this phase there is satisfactory symptom control and normal motor activity is possible, unlike the OFF phase in which symptoms reappear with impaired motor function). On the other hand, a greater impact on gait and basic activities of daily living will be triggered where involved. Finally, people should be instructed and educated in the use of technical aids and adaptations which will enable them to perform better and correctly in basic activities of daily living. In addition, environmental modifications play a very important role in this phase, which allow for a more beneficial environment for the person.

-   Phase IV: In this phase the progression of the disease and the affectation of the person is already more advanced, therefore, it is necessary to maintain and stimulate motor skills. In addition, it is important to train caregivers and/or relatives on the assistance that the person should receive, such as postural changes, fall prevention, transfers, the appearance of trophic changes in the skin and advice on support products.

-   Phase V: Finally, in this last stage the person presents a much more advanced degree of dysmobility, the person tends to spend more time in bed, so treatment should focus on educating and training family members and caregivers on the required postural changes, mobilisations, warning signs and advice on support products. On the other hand, it is important to stimulate the person cognitively in order to slow down cognitive decline.

It is important to highlight that the interventions are different for each person in each of the phases, it is necessary to emphasise the requirements in a personal way, as not all users evolve in the same way (Gómez et al., 2020).

RECOMMENDATIONS ON INTERVENTION STRATEGIES FOR THE TREATMENT OF PEOPLE WITH PARKINSON'S DISEASE BASED ON WHAT HAS BEEN GATHERED THROUGH SCIENTIFIC EVIDENCE.

Proposed Intervention Strategy

As evidenced by a thorough review of each of the studies used in this seminar and research, in addition to the recent literature review related to Parkinson's disease treatment and intervention, it is possible to put forward a proposal for intervention, which is important to consider:

The aim of occupational therapy in Parkinson's disease is to ensure that the affected person is as autonomous and independent as possible, in order to improve and maintain their quality of life. Based on this, it is important to consider the individual needs that characterise each of the users; therefore, an intervention proposal can only be established from the generality of the pathology, without considering more specific factors such as the general state and evolution of the pathology itself in each subject and the personal circumstances of each one.

The following proposal is based on the division of the different activities required in the 5 stages of Parkinson's Disease, as determined by the Hoehn and Yahr scale. Before carrying out any type of intervention, it is necessary to be able to establish a differential diagnosis of P.D. or which are the excluding criteria that are characteristic of the pathology, in addition to carrying out individualised assessments to know the needs and disabilities with which the different users arrive individually; in addition to this, the use of standardised assessments should be considered that allow the intervention to be validated and to be able to carry out re-evaluations, according to the evolution of the disease, using the immediate context, as a therapeutic means to maintain the person's independence for as long as possible.

In order for the intervention to be beneficial for the person, work should be carried out mainly in the person's home or in the place where they spend most of their time, as this is where they will spend most of their time, so that environmental modifications can be made if necessary to maintain the person's independence. When intervening in each of the stages of P.E., pharmacological treatment should be considered together with the non-pharmacological treatment of the multidisciplinary team (kinesiology, speech therapy, among others).

MINSAL Clinical Guideline 2010, Parkinson's Disease Initial Stage (H & Y: 0 to 2)	Proposal of strategies Seminarians Universidad de Playa Ancha
Early assessment and identification of problems related to movement disorders.	Assess and identify movement disorders and the problems they cause for the person's occupational performance through fine and gross motor assessments.
Maintain and prevent the deterioration of processing, communication and social interaction skills.	Assess and identify the problems presented by the person and their environment as a result of the disease. Encourage social participation within the community, through networks. Encourage the reinforcement of cognitive functions.

Encourage the participation of the user with P.E. in programmes designed to improve occupational participation in meaningful activities of basic daily living (ADLB) and instrumental activities of daily living (IADL) as appropriate.	Encourage the participation of the person with P.E. in meaningful programme sessions in all occupational areas performed and considered by the person (work, ADL, leisure and free time, education) as appropriate, through occupational activities similar or equal to their daily activities.
Prevent postural deficiencies, gait and transfer deficiencies.	Improve strategies to support movement and mobility in the community to provide greater independence and autonomy.
Prevent and treat postural instability as appropriate (mainly stage 2).	Maintain postural control in activities and performance in their occupations, through strategies (internal and external) of postural corrections and environmental adaptations. Using physical conditioning activities through structured and sequenced exercises through music.

Use movement strategies throughout the course of the disease.	Improve postural hygiene through energy-saving techniques and joint protection techniques that allow the person to use less energy and thus avoid muscle fatigue.
Educating patients, families and carers.	Educate patients, relatives and caregivers about the disease, preventions and reconditioning that must be carried out to maintain the person's independence.
Modality of individual and group intervention, depending on the therapeutic environment or context that allows it.	Working in group activities gives the person the opportunity to interact with peers and share experiences.
Recommended sessions: 5 sessions per year.	Recommended sessions: 24 sessions per year.
Prevention of caregiver overload	Strengthen protection strategies aimed at the caregiver in order to avoid caregiver syndrome.

MINSAL Clinical Guideline 2010, Parkinson's Disease Intermediate Stage (H & Y 3 and 4)	Proposal of strategies Seminarians Universidad de Playa Ancha
Stimulation of motor, processing, communication and interaction skills.	Identify problems in the execution of activities of daily living, productivity and leisure time. To favour social interaction and communication of the person in groups of P.E. patients and within the community, avoiding social abandonment. Maintain cognitive functions, with varying degrees of difficulty in terms of activities connecting cognitive and motor strategies within a group or individual sequence.
Prevention of falls	Identification of the new condition of the person's performance and participation, favouring autonomy and independence, through external strategies and environmental modifications within the home, work and community.
Assess and identify problems related to movement disorders.	Making of orthoses and adaptations. Maintain occupational performance in meaningful activities. Through challenging activities that destabilise postural control.

Modality of care: Individual and family sessions. Home and community visits.	Facilitating the generation of self-help groups. Emphasis on processes in a community context. Maintenance of support networks. Assess performance issues in social and work contexts for physical and social intervention.
Evidence of elements of caregiver overload.	Restructuring of life routines in favour of the maintenance of the person and his/her family members in activities of interest, avoiding the loss of participation in social and community instances of all family members, and thus avoiding the loss of independence within their activities and occupations.
Recommended sessions: 10 sessions per year.	Recommended sessions: 48 sessions per year.
MINSAL Clinical Guideline 2010, Parkinson's Disease Advanced Stage (H & Y: 4 to 5)	Proposal for strategies Seminarians Universidad de Playa Ancha

Assessment of the person's occupational performance (use of a suggested guideline that can be answered by the caregiver).	Assessment of occupational performance in different areas, specifically basic activities of daily living.
Determine critical areas.	Determine the most affected areas in the person, in order to carry out appropriate training with the caregiver.
Instruct on how to conserve energy in order to be able to perform some ABVD.	Re-educate on energy-saving techniques to optimally realise the remaining areas of occupation.
Treat at home with an exercise regime, taking into account age, cognitive impairment, multiple disorders and medication.	Environmental adaptation, in terms of: Food utensils. Costumes. Displacement and Transfers. Common areas within the home (bedroom, kitchen, bathroom, corridors, etc.).

Ensure proper management of movement and position	Educate the caregiver on the correct positioning of the person according to the normal postural control mechanism.
Avoid falls.	Training of assistance in activities of daily living, favouring as much independence as possible (collaboration, choice in certain steps of the task).
Structuring of life routines, providing leisure and free time for the caregiver. Use of family and community support networks.	Emphasis of the intervention on the caregiver, for the management of the affected person in favour of the quality of life of the family group.
Prevention of injuries due to caregiver overload, postural education, environmental management, use of bars, transfer elements, adaptations in bathrooms, bedrooms, etc.	Reassessment of caregiver overload (Zarit). Individual sessions, family sessions and home visits.

Recommended sessions: 10 sessions per year.	Recommended sessions: 96 sessions per year.

Table 10: Intervention Strategies Recommendations Guide.

Finally, in 3 of the 10 articles analysed, they refer to the importance of individualised and personalised interventions which can consolidate the relationship between client and therapist. But at the same time the results indicate the importance of promoting group sessions in parallel with individual sessions in a complementary way, since group sessions facilitate the participation and motivation of patients to achieve certain changes in behaviour; since this experience has shown that group therapy is very suitable for patients with this type of chronic degenerative diseases who are easily dragged into depression and social isolation. The group provides a supportive environment and facilitates peer interactions. In addition, interventions addressing motor and functional problems should also be accompanied by group sessions which improve socialisation, motivation, interpersonal and family relationships, as well as self-esteem and a better understanding of the disease.

The work of Occupational Therapy is fundamental to carry out an optimal and complete intervention in the treatment of Parkinson's Disease, as it allows the person to cope with the disease in a more balanced way, allowing them to have a better quality of life. It is considered fundamental for the treatment to set objectives centred on the needs and wishes of each user, taking into account the stage of the disease and, as the disease evolves, the activities are modified or adapted according to the skills and abilities that the patient retains. This is why it is complex to contrast the effectiveness of the results of the treatment carried out in each study, as each of them works with a specific focus according to the needs of the study population. Several factors are involved in the results of scientific studies, such as the duration of treatment, number of patients included in the study, assessments and guidelines applied, so, in order to have a better comparison and analysis between them, these factors should be replicated in each study to obtain a more homogeneous analysis and concretely determine the effectiveness of the treatment. It is considered in several of the selected studies that it is important and necessary to work with a multidisciplinary team for treatment, including for example occupational therapists, physiotherapists, neurologists, psychologists, among others, as well as complementing with pharmacological treatment to achieve optimal rehabilitation. Thus taking into account in some cases the effectiveness of occupational therapy in people with Parkinson's disease, where an improvement in quality of life is reflected, as the person achieves greater independence in activities of daily living, so there are benefits, however, not all studies analyzed conclude that the results are significant, which is why there is evidence of a lack of reliability and quality in these studies.

The following are excerpts from the main articles analysed.
"Recommendations for the management of patients with disease. National Experts' Consensus." Avello, R.; Benavides, O.; Chana, P.; Cueto, G.; Cerda A.; Fernández, R.; Jara, R.; Juri, C.; Klapp, C.; Kunstmann, C.; Tapia, j.; Tirapegui, J.

Parkinson's disease (PD) is a progressive neurodegenerative disease with a high impact on sufferers and their families. In 2010, the Chilean Health System included P.S. in the explicit Health guarantees, and clinical guidelines were developed for the diagnosis and treatment of P.S. We reviewed the guidelines for the diagnosis and treatment of P.S. published in the world literature, in order to adapt them to the reality of our country from the perspective of a national group of experts.

2.1.1.   "A Survey of Current Occupational Therapy Practice for Parkinson's Disease in the United Kingdom." Deane, K.; Ellis-Hill, C.; Dekker, K.; Davies, P.; Clarke. C

Little is known about the current nature of occupational therapy practice for Parkinson's disease in the UK. The study aimed to document this to inform plans for a future multicentre randomised controlled trial.

Two hundred and forty-two occupational therapists treating people with Parkinson's disease were sent a questionnaire on demographics, service organisation and therapy content. One hundred and sixty-nine occupational therapists (70%) responded. They had worked with people with Parkinson's disease for a median of 6 years and personally treated a median of 15 people with Parkinson's disease annually. The majority (86%) were at senior grade or above; 87% worked in the National Health Service and 12% in social services. Forty percent worked in specialist Parkinson's disease clinics. Most (79%) felt they needed more specialised postgraduate training.

2.1.2.   "Effectiveness of Occupational Therapy in Parkinson's disease: study protocol for a randomized controlled trial". Sturkenboom, I.; Graff, M.; Borm, G.; Adang, E.; Nijhusis-van der Sander, M.; Bloem, B.; Munneke, M.

Given current changes in health care, being able to obtain and use research evidence to support work-related, therapeutic treatment has become increasingly important. The purpose of this study was to synthesise the available evidence on the effectiveness of Occupational Therapy related treatments for people with Parkinson's Disease. A meta-analysis was conducted to achieve this synthesis. The results reveal small to moderate positive effects of intervention on outcomes related to clients' abilities and skills, as well as for outcomes related to function during activities and tasks. Limitations in the research reviewed for this meta-analysis may have resulted in an underestimation of treatment effects Occupational therapists can use the results of this meta-analysis to communicate with clients about the potential benefits of participating in Occupational Therapy.

2.1.3.   "Physiotherapy and Occupational Therapy vs No Therapy in Mild to Moderate Parkinson Disease." Clarke, C.; Patel, S.; Ives, N.; Rick,

C.; Dowling, F.; Woolley, R.; Wheatley. K.; Sackley, C.

Parkinson's disease (PD) causes problems with activities of daily living (ADLs) that are only partially treated with medication and occasionally surgery. Despite treatment, patients develop intractable motor problems, such as falls, mental health problems and other non-motor symptoms. Physiotherapy (PT) and Occupational Therapy (OT) are traditionally used later in the disease. However, service provision varies widely, with some centres involving physiotherapists and occupational therapists from diagnosis, while other areas have no specialist services. Cochrane reviews of PT for P.E. found small but significant effects on motor function but not on quality of life. A Cochrane review of O.T. found insufficient evidence of effectiveness. Previous trials with both therapies were small with short-term follow-up. Despite this lack of evidence, the UK National Institute for Health and Care Effectiveness guidelines, while acknowledging these shortcomings and recommending further trials, stated that all patients should have access to both therapies. The REHAB PD trial was designed to evaluate the clinical effectiveness and cost-effectiveness of individualised PT and O.T. in patients with P.P. The design of the current trial was informed by the pilot study of O.T. in P.P.

2.1.4.   "The impact of Occupational Therapy in Parkinson 's disease: a randomized controlled feasibility study." Sturkenboom, I.; Graff, M.; Borm, G.; Veenhuizen, Y.; Bloem, B.; Munneke, M.; Nijhusis-van der Sander, M.

The aim of this scientific study is "To assess the feasibility of a randomised trial involving the process and potential impact of Occupational Therapy in Parkinson's Disease"; the process and outcome were evaluated quantitatively and qualitatively in a multicentre, randomised, controlled, exploratory trial three months after the start of the trial; among the participants evaluated were 43 P.D. patients living in the community with difficulties in their activities of daily living, their primary caregivers, and 7 occupational therapists. Treatment was carried out for ten weeks within the home of each patient in the treatment group according to the Dutch guidelines for Occupational Therapy in Parkinson's Disease, while the control group did not receive any treatment during this period of time.

Process evaluation measured accrual, dropout, intervention delivery and protocol adherence. The primary patient outcomes assessed daily functioning: Canadian Occupational Performance Measure (COPM) and Motor and Process Skills Assessment. The primary outcome for caregivers was caregiver burden: Zarit Burden Inventory. Participants' perspectives on the intervention were explored through questionnaires and in-depth interviews.

2.1.5.   "Physical Therapy and Occupational Therapy in Parkinson 's disease." Radder, D.; Sturkenboom, I.; Nimwegen, M.; Keus, S.; Bloem, B.; Vries, N.

Current medical treatment is only partially effective in controlling the symptoms of Parkinson's disease. As part of comprehensive multidisciplinary care, physiotherapy and occupational therapy aim to help people with Parkinson's disease to cope with the consequences of their disease in daily activities. In this narrative review, we address the limitations that people with Parkinson's disease may encounter despite optimal medical treatment, and clarify the unique and shared approaches that physiotherapists and occupational therapists can apply to address these limitations.

2.1.6.   "The Benefits of Group Occupational Therapy for Patients With Parkinson's Disease." Gauthier, L.; Dalziel, S.; Gauthier, S.

Medical treatment of idiopathic Parkinson's disease. The disease has improved the quality of life and increased survival of patients with Parkinson's disease. However, as the disease progresses, impairments in activities of daily living occur. One clinic initiated a trial for a group rehabilitation programme to maintain the functional status of these patients. The research protocol consisted of a pre-treatment assessment, randomisation to experimental or control groups, and post-treatment assessments after therapy, at 6 months and 1 year. Results showed that subjects in the experimental treated group maintained their functional status after 1 year, demonstrated a significant cannot decrease in bradykinesia, and perceived a significant improvement in their psychological well-being. This study confirms the value of a group Occupational Therapy approach and its benefits for functional independence, for the improvement of physical and motor symptoms, and the quality of life of people with Parkinson's disease.

2.1.7.   "Enabling Functional Independence in Parkinson's Disease: Update on Occupational Therapy Intervention." Ashwini, K.; OTR, EdD.

Motor impairment and functional limitations are known sequelae of Parkinson's disease. Occupational Therapy (OT) is recognised as an important adjunct to pharmacological management. This critical review provides an update on the effectiveness of OT. Eight studies were included in the review, three on occupational therapy task-related training, two on functional training with external cues and three on OT as part of interdisciplinary treatment. Due to the lack of level I studies, it is difficult to conclusively determine the effect of O.T. However, there is evidence to suggest that the treatment produces improvements in motor and quality of life over the duration of therapy. Implications for future studies and practice are discussed.

2.1.8.   "Measuring the impact of Parkinson's disease: An Occupational Therapy perspective. Gaudet, P.

Parkinson's disease is a common neurodegenerative disorder that affects more than 100,000 Canadians. With advances in medical and surgical treatments, clients are living longer and fuller lives. However, as the disease progresses, people with Parkinson's continue to face a variety of deficits in occupational performance. Although this is the domain of occupational therapists, very little is described in the literature on Parkinson's-related occupational therapy. This scientific study addresses this gap by describing these deficits and the current measurement tools that can be used to assess the impact on people living with Parkinson's disease. Although several tools are cited, three tools are recommended for an Occupational Therapy assessment of individuals with Parkinson's Disease: the Canadian Occupational Performance Measure.

2.1.9.   "A Process Evaluation of a Home-Based Occupational Therapy Intervention for Parkinson's Patients and Their Caregivers Performed Alongside a Randomized Controlled Trial" Sturkenboom, I.; Nijhusis-van der Sander, M.; Graff, M.

Objective: To evaluate the fidelity, treatment delivery and experiences of an occupational therapy intervention in Parkinson's disease, to identify factors affecting intervention delivery and benefits. Design: Mixed methods in conjunction with a randomised controlled trial. Subjects: These included 124 patients with Parkinson's disease living at home and their primary caregivers (recipients) and 18 occupational therapists. Intervention: 10-week home-based intervention according to the Dutch guidelines for Occupational Therapy in Parkinson's Disease. Main measures: Data were collected on intervention dose, protocol process, treatment content (fidelity), strategies offered and delivered (treatment enactment) and recipients' experiences. Therapists' experiences were collected through case note analysis and focus group interviews. Results: The mean intervention dose was 9.3 (SD 2.3) hours. Mean adherence to the protocol process was high (93%; SD 9%), however, the intervention did not (fully) address the target for 268 of 617 treatment goals. The frequencies of strategies offered and delivered appeared similar, apart from "use other tools and materials", which showed a drop from 279 advised to 149 used. Recipients were generally satisfied with the intervention (mean score 8 out of 10). Therapists noted positive or negative influencing factors on both process and benefits: the research context, the socio-political context of health care, recipients' personal and contextual factors, and therapists' competence.

BIBLIOGRAPHICAL REFERENCES

- Alburquerque, D., Aránguiz, R., Baldwin, N., Benavides, O., De la Cerda, A., Curinao, X., Tapia, S. (2010). Parkinson's disease. Retrieved from http://cetram.org/wp/wp-content/uploads/2013/11/libroPark.pdf

- Agorreta, E; Urteaga, G; Fernández, R (2015). Occupational therapy intervention in users with neurological pathology and/or physical dysfunction. Retrieved from http://www.revistatog.com/num22/pdfs/revision5.pdf

- Ambrosio, L., Portillo M., Rodríguez, C., Rojo, J. & Martínez, P. (2019). Influencing factors when Living with Parkinson's Disease: A cross-sectional study.

- Arroyo, M; Finkel, L. (2013). Dependence and social impact of Parkinson's disease.

- Arredondo-Blanco, K., Zerón-Martínez, R., Rodríguez-Violante, M. and Cervantes-Arriaga, A. (2018). Brief historical overview of Parkinson's Disease 200 years after its description. Gaceta Medica de México 154:719-726. DOI: 10.24875/GMM.18003702.

- Ashwini, K.; OTR, EdD. (2010). Enabling Functional Independence in Parkinson's Disease: Update on Occupational Therapy Intervention.

- Avello, R.; Benavides, O.; Chana, P.; Cueto, G.; Cerda A.; Fernández, R.; Jara, R.; Juri, C.; Klapp, C.; Kunstmann, C.; Tapia, J.; Tirapegui, J. (2012). National Expert Consensus: recommendations for the management of patients with Parkinson's disease.

- Berganzo, K., Tijero B., González-Eizaguirre, A., Somme, J., Lezcano, E., Gabilondo, I., Fernández, M., Zarranz and J., Gómez-Esteban, J (2016). Non-motor and motor symptoms in Parkinson's Disease and their relationship with quality of life and different clinical subgroups. Neurology, 2016; 31(9): 585-591. Doi: 10.1016/j.nrl.2014.10.010.

- Botella, J.; Zamora, A. (2017). Meta-analysis: a methodology for research in education.

- Castillero, O (S/F). What is psychosis? Causes, symptoms and treatment. Psychology and Mind. Retrieved from https://psicologiaymente.com/clinica/psicosis

- Chana, P; Parkinson's Disease (2010); 1st edition; Cetram, Usach. Retrieved from: https://books.google.cl/books?id=7PdsxtAtfagC&pg=PA86&dq=parkinson+and+occupational+therapy&hl=en-419&sa=X&ved=0ahUKEwiNo8XUu-jmAhXPILkGHVrECr4Q6AEIMTAB#v=onepage&q=parkinson%20and%20occupational%20therapy&f=false

- Clarke, C.; Patel, S.; Ives, N.; Rick, C.; Dowling, F.; Woolley, R.; Wheatley.K.; Sackley, C. (2016). Physiotherapy and Occupational Therapy v/s No therapy in mild to moderate Parkinson's disease.

- International Classification of Functioning, Disability and Health [ICF] (2001). Definition of Functioning. Retrieved from: https://apps.who.int/iris/bitstream/handle/10665/43360/9241545445_spa. pdf?sequence=1

- Deane, K.; Ellis-Hill, C.; Dekker, K.; Davies, P.; Clarke. C. (2016). A survey of current Occupational Therapy practice for Parkinson's disease in the United Kingdom.

- Dixon L, Duncan D, Johnson P, Kirkby L, O'Connell H, Taylor H. (2017) Occupational therapy for patients with Parkinson's disease. Retrieved from http://www.sld.cu/galerias/pdf/sitios/rehabilitacionadulto/terapia_ocupacio nal_for_patients_with_parkinson's_disease.pdf

- World Federation of Occupational Therapists [WFOT] (2004). Definition of Occupational Therapy. Retrieved from: http://www.terapeutas-ocupacionales.com/2012/09/definiciones-de-terapia-ocupacional.html

- Figueira, L. (2012). Pramipexole in the Treatment of Parkinson's Disease, 14(3): 111-119.

- Gauthier, L.; Dalziel, S.; Gauthier, S. (2020). The benefits of group Occupational Therapy for patients with Parkinson's disease.

- Hernández R, Fernández C & Baptista P. (1997). Research

methodology. Retrieved from: https://www.uv.mx/personal/cbustamante/files/2011/06/Metodologia-de- la-Investigaci%C3%83%C2%B3n_Sampier

- Gómez-Chavarín, M., Roldan-Roldan, G., Morales-Espinosa, R., Pérez- Soto, G. and Torner-Aguilar, C. (2012). Pathophysiological mechanisms involved in Parkinson's disease. Archivos de Neurociencia Instituto Nacional de Neurología y Neurocirugía, 17(1): 26-34.

- Hernández R, Fernández C & Baptista P. (2014). Research methodology. Retrieved from: https://www.esup.edu.pe/descargas/dep_investigacion/Metodologia%20d e%20la%20investigaci%20la%20investigaci%20C3%B3n%205ta%20Edici%20C3%B3n.pdf

- Herrera S. (2014). Alteraciones emocionales en la fase inicial de la Enfermedad de Parkinson. junio 2014, de Universidad de Salamanca Sitio web:https://gredos.usal.es/bitstream/handle/10366/123405/TFM_Her rera Z%C3%BA%C3%B1igaSG_alteraciones.pdf?sequence=1&isAllowed =y

- Hurtado, F., Cárdenas, M. A., Cárdenas, F. and León, L. A. (2016). Parkinson's Disease: Etiology, Treatments and Preventive Factors.

- Ibáñez, V; Modesto, V. (2005). Introduction to evidence-based medicine.

- Jansa, J.; Aragon, A. (2015). Living with Parkinson's and emerging role of Occupational Therapy.

- Leiva, A; Martínez, M; Troncoso, C; Nazar, G; Petermann, F; Celis, C. (2019). Chile leads the Latin American ranking of Parkinson's disease prevalence. Rev. méd. Chile vol.147 no.4. Retrieved from https://scielo.conicyt.cl/scielo.php?script=sci_arttext&pid=S0034-98872019000400535

- Málaga, G; Neira-Sánchez, E. (2018). Evidence-based medicine, its evolution 25 years after its dissemination, promoting a scientific, caring, loving and humane clinical practice.

- Ministry of Health [MINSAL] (2010). Guía Clínica Enfermedad de Parkinson. Retrieved from:https://www.minsal.cl/portal/url/item/955578f79a0cef2ae0 4001011f01678a.

- Micheli, F. (2006). Parkinson's Disease and Related Disorders. Buenos Aires, Argentina: Editorial Médica Panamericana S.A.

- Ministry of Health [MINSAL] (2016). Guía Clínica AUGE Enfermedad de Parkinson, Tratamiento no Farmacológico de Rehabilitación. Retrieved from:http://www.bibliotecaminsal.cl/wp/wpcontent/uploads/2016/04/G PC-EP-Tratamiento-no-farmacologico-EP-final-17-03-2016.pdf

- Ministry of Health [MINSAL] (2010). Parkinson's disease clinical guidelines. Retrieved from https://www.minsal.cl/portal/url/item/955578f79a0cef2ae04001011f01 678 a.pdf

- Radder, D.; Sturkenboom, I.; Nimwegen, M.; Keus, S.; Bloem, B.; Vries, N. (2017). Physical therapy and occupational therapy in Parkinson's disease.

- Rodríguez-Violante, M., Cervantes-Arriaga, A. and Arellano-Reynoso, A. (2014). Deep brain stimulation in Parkinson's disease: Importance of a multidisciplinary team.

- Sáenz de Pipaón, I. and Larumbe, R. (2001). Neurodegenerative diseases programme. ANALES Sis San Navarra, 24(3): 49-76.

- Sturkenboom, I.; Nijhusis-van der Sander, M.; Graff, M. (2015). A process evaluation of a home-based occupational therapy intervention for Parkinson's patients and their caregivers performed alongside a randomized controlled trial.

- Sturkenboom, I.; Graff, M.; Borm, G.; Adang, E.; Nijhusis-van der Sander, M.; Bloem, B.; Munneke, M. (2013). Effectiveness of occupational therapy in Parkinson's disease: study for a randomized controlled trial.

- Simó, S. (2015). Occupational therapy from a critical paradigm. Retrieved from http://www.revistatog.com/mono/num7/mono7.pdf
- Sturkenboom, I.; Graff, M.; Borm, G.; Veenhuizen, Y.; Bloem, B.; Munneke, M.; Nijhusis-van der Sander, M. (2012). The impact of occupational therapy in Parkinson's disease: a randomized controlled feasibility study.
- Zarranz, J. (2013). Neurology. Barcelona, Spain: Elsevier

Table of Contents

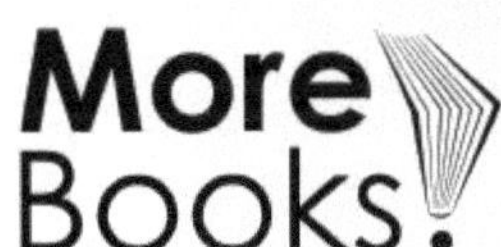

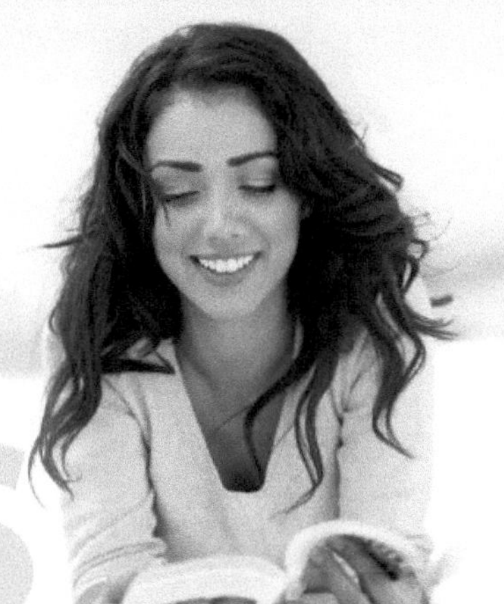

yes

I want morebooks!

Buy your books fast and straightforward online - at one of world's fastest growing online book stores! Environmentally sound due to Print-on-Demand technologies.

Buy your books online at
www.morebooks.shop

Kaufen Sie Ihre Bücher schnell und unkompliziert online – auf einer der am schnellsten wachsenden Buchhandelsplattformen weltweit! Dank Print-On-Demand umwelt- und ressourcenschonend produzi ert.

Bücher schneller online kaufen
www.morebooks.shop

info@omniscriptum.com
www.omniscriptum.com

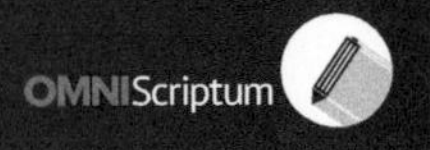